Hospital Survival Guide:
A Physical Therapy Perspective

Hospital Survival Guide:
A Physical Therapy Perspective

Ronald M. Wild, PT

This book is dedicated to all those who have loved ones struggling with illness and difficult times. It is dedicated to all of my family members who have been there for me every day of my life—especially my mother, whom I could not begin to thank for all her love and support.

Contents

Introduction

A hospital stay can be an intimidating and overwhelming experience for patients and families. There is nothing more stressful than having a loved one fall ill. The hospital environment is not always friendly. Multiple issues can be happening simultaneously that are not easily understandable. The intent of this manual is to give patients and family members a concise guide to navigate the hospital experience. It is meant to help minimize the stress associated with a hospital stay by giving some simple explanations, descriptions and suggestions. This manual is not intended to be an all-inclusive reference guide. It is my sincere hope that this small publication assists you in avoiding some major pitfalls and makes the hospital experience more manageable. It should help direct you through the basic inquiry process and get you started.

My first attempt at this manual ended with a final product that was well over one hundred pages and just too cumbersome for patients and families to use as a quick reference guide. Therefore, in this iteration, I have eliminated a lot of the details as they are easily and quickly found with a little research. My goal with this manual is to direct your ability to ask the appropriate questions by giving you some basic information, references, and thought processes. Obviously, without being there, I cannot predict many of the specific events and questions that arise with each individual hospital stay. Take the information provided here and use your judgment in its application.

This manual is focused on the hospital setting; however, there is some crossover relevance to other health-care settings. Although there are some differences in the various settings, much of the information does not change from hospital to skilled nursing facility (extended-care facility), to acute rehabilitation hospital, to long-term acute care hospital, and so on.

Being in the hospital can be overwhelming for several reasons. First, the emotion involved with having a loved one in the hospital can cloud logical thinking. Second, the amount of information being thrown at you is significant and usually occurs in a very brief period. Typically, when the doctor walks in the room and gives you all the information, he or she must impart it in the shortest time possible. Third, if you don't have a medical background, you are learning an entirely new language. As with any industry, health care has a language all its own. Fortunately, in the age of the Internet and mobile phones, it is easy to become fluent quite rapidly. Just take each of your questions one at a time, and you will be surprised how quickly everything begins to make sense. When I attended physical therapy school, before the explosion of the Internet, I had to use the old-fashioned medical encyclopedia. Things have become much more convenient since then with the availability of online resources. I need to stress that this manual will not answer all your questions. It is just a starting point. My assumption is that you have had very little exposure to hospitalization and health care.

Throughout this manual I use the term "clinician" frequently. It is a general term referring to health-care professionals who provide patient care. This can mean doctors, nurses, therapists, nurse practitioners, physician assistants, and the like. The other term I use often is "hospitalist." I use this to refer to the attending physician. This is the doctor who coordinates all the care while you are in the hospital. Basically, this is the primary-care physician for your time in the hospital. Obviously, each health-care facility has its own policies, procedures, and individual ways of doing things. Job titles, job duties, and procedural methods will vary, but the general idea behind each section in this manual remains the same. I have limited the use of medical terminology to scenarios in which knowing the term will facilitate communication with hospital staff. Take a deep breath and continue reading. Do not just go along without asking questions. Be an active participant in the process. You are more than capable of managing this situation with a little knowledge and effort.

One

The Perspective of This Manual

I am a physical therapist with almost twenty years of hospital and specialty hospital experience. This experience includes being a staff physical therapist and holding various administrative positions. Therefore, as implied in the title, this manual is from the perspective of the discipline associated with mobility. When using the term "mobility," I am specifically referring to the ability to move in bed, sit on the edge of the bed, stand up, walk, and climb stairs—in other words, all the activities that people will need to perform in their daily lives once they leave the hospital. This is referred to in the hospital as activities of daily living (ADLs).

I am not a physician, a nurse, or a pharmacist. I cannot prescribe medications. While I do not address any specific medications, I do address the overall potential impact of medications on a patient's mobility and independence. It is also important to have a basic understanding about what is happening with patient medication, as this can have an effect on the patient in many ways.

There are several advantages to looking at a hospital stay from the perspective of a physical therapist. Typically, functional independence (being able to stand, walk, climb stairs, and perform daily activities without assistance) is the ultimate goal prior to going home. For the most part, everything else needs to be going well for the patients to progress with therapy. They need to be medically stable and have a level of alertness and cognition that allows them to follow some basic commands. I see patients daily with the sole focus of determining mobility improvement from day to day. As a physical therapist, I assess mobility progress as well as things that may be impeding progress. I do not prescribe any type of medical treatment (beyond the mobility plan of care) and therefore am not invested in what is being prescribed either in terms of medications or procedures. My only objective is to help patients attain their maximum level of independence with regard to mobility. My job is to assess patients' ability to function at home and in the community. If they are unable to do so, I must determine both the barriers and the underlying causes of those barriers. For example, let's suppose a patient is confused and unable to follow commands to stand, walk, and perform basic ADLs safely. Is this confusion due to medications, a stroke, or the exacerbation of a previously undiagnosed dementia? Even though actual diagnoses of these conditions lie with the physician, my experience is that of advancing patients' mobility independence so that they can return home safely, as well as identifying and overcoming barriers to that outcome.

Two

Recognize Stress in Yourself

Obviously, having a loved one in the hospital is one of the most stress-ful situations imaginable. It is normal to experience stress. Stress has a tendency to make even minor issues or problems seem major. It is important to recognize this when you are interacting with people and making decisions. In the hospital, things don't always go exactly as you expect. When issues arise, be sure to maintain a focus on the big picture and maintain perspective when handling problems. Ideally, you want to find someone to speak with during this process who can give you an objective perspective on the situation. This could be a friend or family member who has a calm demeanor, someone who you can bounce ideas off. This person should be able to help you differentiate the important issues from those that only seem important in the moment.

Three

Be Nice to Staff

Always be pleasant when dealing with hospital staff. It is a natural human tendency to gravitate to people we enjoy being around. You want staff to feel comfortable approaching you. Be friendly, smile, and act as though these people have the life of your loved one in their hands—because they do. Being friendly to staff members and encouraging them to approach you with both positive and negative information alike can help keep you updated on the patient's status. Whenever possible, spend a short amount of time getting to know each staff member after the admission process. Be sincere in your interactions. This short time investment can pay off exponentially. If you are demanding, complaining, and always asking staff to run insignificant errands and make accommodations, this will not encourage them to check on you more frequently than is necessary.

However, note that being personable and approachable does not imply settling for a lower level of care or ignoring issues relating to patient care. If issues do arise, as they inevitably will, do not be afraid to address them. Seek to understand the situation first. Do not be accusatory. Do not jump to conclusions. Do not exaggerate the importance of the issue. Minimize drama. A hospital is like many other businesses from the standpoint that there are many different types of employees with many different levels of competency and different work ethics. If you have already established a good relationship with staff members, they will typically bend over backward to accommodate you. If there is an issue that does not get handled by speaking with staff members directly, you can go to the charge nurse on the floor. Don't elevate issues that are not important. Stick to patient-care issues. Each hospital will have different titles and chains of command. Your issue should be resolved prior to the end of the current shift during which you address that issue. If the charge nurse does not address the issue in a reasonable amount of time, elevate the issue to the house supervisor, the chief nursing officer, the hospitalist, or the hospital administration.

Four

Keep a Journal

Be sure to keep some type of journal. It can be a paper or an electronic one. I prefer paper. Do not use individual pieces of paper and place them in a folder at a later time. They will get lost. Divide the journal into two sections. In the first section, keep a log of what happens over the course of each day. Don't get carried away with all the details. Just include the important things that happened that day and updates from physicians, nurses, and other health-care professionals. Include who you spoke with, their titles, and the information they imparted. Have a second section to write down any questions you have. This will allow you to have the questions available when the physician or other appropriate professional enters the room. It is very common to have multiple questions after you have had a discussion with a provider, often after you have had time to process the information they have given you. Write down your questions immediately for the next time you see that provider. This will also help you track and organize the information as your questions get answered.

Begin by asking the nurses to answer your questions. If the nurse does not know the answer, he or she should refer you to the appropriate professional. If this individual refers you to someone else, be sure to write that person's name, title, and contact information next to the question. The cardinal rule is to have the journal accessible at all times.

Use the following approach when having questions answered. I will reiterate this process in the discharge section as well:

1. Ask the question.
2. Listen to the answer.
3. When you think you understand, respond as follows: "If I understand correctly, you said (repeat back to the person what you believe he or she told you)."
4. Write what the individual said in your journal immediately.

This process will dramatically reduce miscommunication.

Five

Ask a Lot of Questions

I encourage you to ask a lot of questions. In the beginning, if you have no health-care experience or background, it will seem that there is an overwhelming amount of information being thrown at you. Eventually, with persistence, you will find that as you get one question answered, it gives you the ability to ask several more directed questions, and the process continues until you are able to get an overall picture of what is happening. Ask that one question that seems ridiculous. That may be the question that gives you the information you need to open the door to understanding everything that is happening. The first few questions are the most difficult. Remember, clinicians are not there just to take care of your loved one; one of their primary responsibilities is to educate you as well. When asking questions, be respectful of the clinicians' time as they have busy schedules. This means having your questions written down and organized to the best of your ability. This is not always possible as hospital stays can be very fluid experiences. Don't be afraid to take sufficient time to get your questions answered but, again, be organized and respectful of their busy schedules.

Be aware that the hospital staff carries out many of their activities based on physician orders. These orders are located in a specific section of the patient chart. They are written by the physician and direct what the physician expects the staff to do. *If you have a conversation with the physician, and the physician tells you he or she is going to have a member of the staff carry out a task, ask if the physician is going to write an order directing that task to be performed. Then, after a reasonable amount of time, check with the nurse to be certain that the doctor did in fact remember to write the order.*

It is a good idea when you first meet with the hospitalist or the nurse to ask what other types of physicians have been or will be consulted and their names. You want to know this as there may be several doctors with the same specialty. You want to know specifically who is going to be on the case. The hospitalist may consult several other physicians who are specialists. Here are a few examples: nephrologist (kidneys), orthopedist, infectious disease (ID), cardiologist, physiatrist (rehabilitation), psychiatrist, neurologist, pulmonologist (lungs), and urologist, as well as various types of surgeons. Knowing which of these specialists has been consulted allows you to direct your questions more appropriately.

Asking about normal bodily functions is always a good place to start when asking questions. Ask about patient nutrition. Ask about bowel and bladder function. Constipation is a concern for anyone who is immobile and/or on pain medication. This can be a serious issue in the hospital. Ask about medications. I cover this topic in greater detail in the medications section below.

Six

Communication in
Health-Care Settings

One of the most likely causes of errors in a hospital situation (and life) is miscommunication. This can occur when a patient is transferred between facilities, between floors or units within a hospital, or even between shifts of employees. Each facility has different processes and procedures. Therefore, the level of communication can vary greatly. It is never a bad idea to remind staff about critical information related to the patient, especially upon admission or moving units. Do not assume all the critical information has been communicated. It is appropriate to remind staff about issues such as medication allergies, limited weight bearing on an extremity (for instance, due to a fracture), blood clots/ deep vein thrombosis (DVT), or any information that might not have been passed along between facilities and staff members. Ask if it would be possible to hang a sign by the bed informing staff of *critical* information, if this has not already been done. Be sure it is important medical/ clinical information. Examples of important information include issues such as the patient having a humeral fracture (broken bone) in the left arm and the surgeon has ordered no weight bearing on that arm or that the patient is allergic to morphine. Again, this must be *critical information* that, if there were to be a mistake concerning, the patient could be harmed. Even though a sign is present, a friendly verbal reminder to staff members who have not yet taken care of the patient is not a bad idea. It is not possible to overcommunicate. As always, be respectful as this is an educated professional. I like to begin with "I'm certain you are already aware."

There is one other issue that applies only in circumstances where there are multiple family members. It is a good idea for the family to get together and choose one spokesperson to give and receive communication on behalf of the entire family. Typically, this will be the medical power of attorney (MPOA) if there is one designated. It is not uncommon for families to have varying points of view on the direction of care. In this case, it is important for families to be responsible for communicating among themselves. Patient care suffers when different family members are giving different instructions to staff. In addition, if several family members are requesting the same information from staff multiple times because they are not communicating among themselves, it takes time from patient care. Have a family meeting and discuss who the official spokesperson is. This does not mean that when other family is visiting, they cannot receive updates. However, any care decisions should go through the spokesperson. Remember that any updates received by any family members should be recorded in the journal.

Seven

Give an Accurate History of the Patient

In all my years of practice, I have never understood one phenomenon that occurs very frequently, and it does not matter how clearly the questions are posed and what clarifications are made. For whatever reason, it is very common for patients and families to overstate how well the patient was doing prior to being hospitalized. Please be certain to give an accurate history of the patient. If the patient has not walked more than fifty feet in the past ten years, do not attempt to conceal this fact. If the patient used a walker or cane before coming to the hospital, be certain to mention this fact. Exaggerating what the patient was able to do, stating what they were doing decades ago (as if it were current information), or filling in information when you are not exactly certain of the facts will make the entire process more frustrating for all involved. Medical staff is not there to judge you. That is not the reason they are asking about the patient's status prior to getting sick. Clinicians are trying to get an accurate baseline so they are able to develop reasonable goals for that individual patient. From a physical therapy standpoint, for example, we inquire about the patient's mobility status immediately prior to becoming sick. If the patient was a crossfit athlete, our goals, approach, and expectations are going to be much more aggressive than someone who would become fatigued by walking twenty feet. I gave this as a therapy-specific example, but the same can be applied when speaking with physicians, nurses, or other health-care professionals. Ultimately, experienced clinicians are going to pick up on any deceptions or exaggerations. Overstating previous abilities or level of health will not motivate therapists to achieve a better outcome. It will merely result in unreasonable and unachievable goals being set and may therefore actually be counterproductive.

Be concise when answering questions. Health histories are sometimes very complex, but do your best to supply only the pertinent information relevant to each question being asked. Disclosing any unique individual tendencies or lifestyles can also sometimes be very helpful. For example, if the patient works a third-shift job and sleeps during the day, this is good for the staff and physician to be aware of as the patient's normal sleep pattern is obviously different than that of most people.

Eight

Changes in Status

This may be one of the most important topics I address in this manual. It is very important to be aware of any sudden changes in the patient's status. For example, sudden lethargy, weakness on one side of the body, sudden onset of confusion, or acute pain/redness/swelling anywhere in the body should be taken very seriously by staff and addressed. Clinicians should already be aware of changes in the patient, but I strongly encourage family to be aware as well. After all, the family typically knows the patient better than any clinician. With the following chart, I am by no means attempting to diagnose your loved one. I am merely providing you a good starting point for discussion. It will be up to the clinical staff to determine what is actually causing these symptoms.

Look Out For	Possible Cause	Possible Follow-up
Sudden weakness, facial droop, foot drop on one side of the body (hemiparesis)	Stroke (cerebral vascular accident—CVA)	CT or MRI of the head
Sudden and pronounced lethargy	Overmedicated, infection, brain involvement; less likely—respiratory	Review medications, check labs for infection, MRI

Look Out For	Possible Cause	Possible Follow-up
	patients with increased carbon dioxide in blood	head, arterial blood gas (ABG) if respiratory involvement
Change in mentation or confusion	Same as above	Same as above
Areas of redness, pain, or swelling in an extremity (arm or leg) that is not otherwise explained	Possible deep vein thrombosis (DVT)	Ultrasound
New rapid breathing or heart rate not due to exertion	Multiple causes	Discuss with physician and nursing staff

Again, this chart is not providing you the tools to diagnose medical conditions. That is the responsibility of the physician. This is only a starting point for conversation with the health-care professionals. These are issues you may encounter that you should make health-care providers aware of. Do not panic if you notice any of the above issues as patients can present with all different types of symptoms in the hospital for a multitude of reasons. Be certain to make sure that clinical staff is aware and that you are getting answers to your questions. In addition, do not assume that because you told one staff member about an issue that he or she has communicated this information to all others. It is best to mention such issues to all appropriate staff including but not limited to physicians, nurses, therapists, physician assistants, and nurse practitioners. Too much communication in this situation is better than not enough. If you have attempted to get answers and are still not confident that the issue has been resolved, this would be an appropriate time to elevate your concerns to supervisors, managers, and administrators.

Nine

Trust but Verify

Please keep in mind that having the initials MD, OT, RN, PT, or RRT after his or her name does not make that person infallible. It has been my experience that older patients, such as of the World War II generation, tend to trust medical staff more blindly than younger generations. If you are uncomfortable with any tests, medications, or treatments, do your own research and speak with your family doctor or neighborhood pharmacist. It is also not a bad idea to ask multiple staff members their opinions. Phrase your question this way when asking staff for an opinion that might be uncomfortable for them to answer: "If it were your family member in this situation, what would you do?" This opens the question to a hypothetical scenario not directly speaking to that situation. This may allow staff to speak more openly.

Ten

Medications

Before I begin this section, I want to emphasize that I am not a physician, nurse, or pharmacist. It is not within my scope of practice to prescribe or recommend medications. I will not be discussing any specific medications or my opinion of certain medications. Despite this, working in a hospital setting for years has shown me the effect that medications can have on a patient's mobility and independence, both positive and negative.

I cannot overemphasize the importance of monitoring the patient's medications. Here is my recommendation regarding how to go about this process.

Start by getting a list of all the medications the patient was taking prior to being admitted to the hospital. Next, ask the nurse for a list of all the medications the patient is currently taking in the hospital. It is your right to request this list. It is referred to as the medication administration record (MAR). Compare both lists. Be aware that hospitals may substitute some medications for others (switching a cheaper generic for a brand-name medication) for cost reasons. Identify any medications that the patient was taking prior to admission that he or she is not currently taking or any new medications the patient is taking now that he or she was not taking prior to admission. You can look online as the drug manufacturers will have a website for each individual medication, including what the drug does and potential side effects. PDR.net is another online reference. Your neighborhood pharmacist can also be a resource, or you can make an appointment with the hospital pharmacist.

Drugs have two names—first the brand name and secondly the generic name. You will need to know the generic names of all the medications for comparison. At first, this will be an intimidating process. Medication names can look like a foreign language. However, the functions of the medications and the side effects are usually relatively easy to understand. Take the time to do this! It may be the most important thing you do in advocating for the patient. Now write down the function of each medication.

After you have identified all medication changes, sit down with the hospitalist or a nurse in whom you have confidence and inquire about all the medication changes you have identified.

- Why were each of these medications added or discontinued?
- What are the most common side effects of each medication added?
- What are the effects of discontinuing any medications the patient was taking at home and is not currently taking?

Write down all information from your research in your journal. As you find the potential side effects of the medications, keep in the back of your mind any changes that may be occurring with the patient. I cannot emphasize enough the importance of doing this. If you get nothing else from this manual, this step alone could be worth your investment. Do your own research on medications. Do not just count exclusively on the expertise of clinicians.

One of the primary reasons to understand changes in medications is that if the patient is experiencing symptoms he or she has not had previously, it could be due to the illness, or it could be an effect of changing medications.

Having a basic understanding of the medications has the added benefit of letting you know conditions that the physicians have identified and are attempting to treat. It will direct your ability to ask pertinent questions and may alert you to issues or medical conditions of which you were previously unaware. It will give you a clearer picture of what is going on overall with the patient.

Finally, I would like to discuss pain medications specifically. They can be a double-edged sword. In some circumstances, they allow patients who are experiencing pain enough relief to participate in therapy and other activities. Pain medications can also cause confusion, lethargy, and constipation, thereby impeding progress in therapy and delaying discharge home. As with all the medications, be sure to ask a lot of questions. Pay special attention to pain medications. Ask the nurse specifically about pain medications, when they were given, and how much was given on the day shift and the prior night shift. If you are noticing confusion or lethargy, be sure to discuss this with the hospitalist.

Eleven

Patient Confusion

It is not uncommon for patients to become confused or disoriented over the course of a hospital stay. There are multiple reasons for this, including medications and trauma to the body and brain. Even though it is not uncommon, this is an issue that needs to be diagnosed and addressed. I highly encourage families to do an objective assessment of the patient's orientation. It is sometimes very difficult for families to be objective in this situation. The family wants the patient to be well, and this often clouds an objective assessment. Confusion can be an issue with a discharge home as it impairs that patient's ability to make good decisions.

Asking the patient, "Do you know where you are?" and receiving an affirmative response is not a valid testing measure.

Ask these questions:

(1) What is your name? Usually, patients will be able to recall their own names. If patients are unable to recall their own names, this is an indicator of profound confusion.
(2) Who am I?
(3) What is today's date?
(4) Do you know where you are? If they do not know, inform them that they are in the hospital. If they do know that they are in the hospital, ask, "Do you recall what happened?"

Wait for the patient to respond to each question. *Do not* give clues or lead the patient. If the patient is unable to answer any of the above questions, give him or her the correct information to fill in the blanks. Repeat this process every time you visit the patient in the hospital. It will allow you to assess improvements in his or her cognition and to assess his or her recall of information you have given the patient on previous visits. Use your journal, and document what you are finding. Track any deficiencies every time you visit.

If the patient is unable to speak for some reason, such as being on a ventilator, go through the above process but stick with yes-or-no questions. In some cases, you may be able to read the patient's lips, but the following process will work well for the times when you are unable to do so. As above, start with "Do you know your name?" Cue the patient to nod yes or no. Tell him or her not to attempt to mouth the words. If you cue the patient to nod yes or no several times and he or she continues to try to mouth words, this may be indicative of confusion. If the patient nods yes to knowing his or her name, follow up with a wrong response. For example, if the patient's actual name is Jack, ask, "Is your name Bob?" Again, be sure to cue the patient to nod if you cannot read his or her lips. If the year is 2016, begin with the question "Is the year 1999?" Continue by asking the correct year, day, month. Do the same with place orientation. "Do you know where you are?" If the patient nods, ask, "Are you at the library?" Continue with questioning as above, and orient the patient as needed.

Understanding a patient's level of cognition is critical. If the patient was living independently prior to hospitalization and is now confused, this is what the hospital will refer to as "a barrier to discharge home." Therefore, it is important to understand the reason (or etiology) for the confusion.

In some cases of confusion, patients are at risk of injuring themselves by pulling on lines or falling, for example; therefore, hospitals may use a variety of devices to prevent injury. These may include mittens, bed alarms, arm/leg restraints, and a variety of other devices that vary by facility.

Confusion is not always profound. Sometimes confusion can be very subtle. It is fairly easy to identify when a patient does not know his or her name, where he or she is, or what happened. That being said, some patients are very adept at hiding even profound confusion. A bigger issue can present itself when the confusion appears only with higher-level thinking and problem solving. For example, the patient may be able to appropriately answer the basic orientation questions above. However, he or she cannot put together the cause and effect of participation in therapy. So someone who was previously active now does not understand that he or she has to participate in therapy in order to get stronger so he or she can go home. You may notice personality changes as well.

Confusion that was not present prior to being hospitalized should be discussed with the physician. He or she should be able to articulate the possible causes of this confusion. This is a good time to ask for a medication review. Did the brain experience a hypoxic (lack of oxygen) event at some point? This may be seen after a cardiac event. Is there a new (acute) process going on (such as a new stroke)? Is there some sort of infectious process? This will be found by reviewing the patient's lab results. Don't be intimidated when clinicians respond with words such as "encephalopathy." Basically that means there is something wrong with the brain. It does not imply a permanent condition. The correct response is to inquire what the cause of the encephalopathy might be.

Twelve

Skin

The skin is the body's protective barrier. It keeps out most infections when it is intact. One of the leading causes of mortality in health-care settings is skin breakdown. This can occur very rapidly for patients who are in a sedated state or who are generally unable to move. Obviously, this is not generally a concern for younger, healthier patients who are mobile. Patients who are older, have circulatory issues, are immobile for any reason, or have skin integrity issues are at a greater risk of skin breakdown and subsequent infection. Body fluids can also exacerbate the breakdown of skin if they are not cleaned regularly. Anytime body fluids are trapped against the skin for a prolonged period of time, the skin can become macerated and break down, leaving that area susceptible to infection. One example is if adult diapers are not frequently changed. The hospital will most likely have some type of process or protocol that involves turning the immobile patient at least every two hours to prevent any one area of skin from bearing weight for an extended period of time. Any kind of bony prominence (area of the body where the bone is not very deep under the surface) is at greater risk of breakdown. Think about the back of the heels, back of the elbows, sacrum (area just above the butt), back of the head, or the scapulae. The sacrum and the heels are especially vulnerable. If the patient meets the above criteria and is not able to move him- or herself in bed, it is a good idea to discuss the process of pressure relief with the nursing staff upon admission.

Thirteen

Mobility

This section is disproportionately long for two reasons. First, this is my field of specialty. Second, this is the focus of many family members, as they feel that once the patient starts moving, his or her health is improving. Mobility is critical for returning patients to their prior levels of function (e.g., bed mobility, standing, walking, and driving). Mobility helps increase circulation, which in turn increases the body's ability to heal. Weight bearing is critical for maintaining the body's core strength.

For patients who have been bedbound for a while, there is a typical progression of mobility. It is fairly intuitive and begins with sitting and then progresses to standing and eventually walking (ambulation). Before patients can stand, they need to have enough trunk strength to sit. Before patients can walk, they need to have the trunk strength to stand. Although this seems to be common sense, it is not uncommon for patients and families to believe that people who are unable to sit may be able to stand or walk. A patient without the trunk stability to sit is generally not going to be able to stand and walk without a significant amount of assistance. First, patients who have been bedbound for an extended period are going to take a few days to get accustomed to sitting in a chair. Thinking about this transition from a purely weight-distribution perspective, when the body is in bed, the weight is distributed over the entire back of the body from head to toes. This is a relatively large surface area. Therefore, the weight on any one area is minimized because of the large area of distribution. Once the patient is sitting in a chair, the weight is primarily placed on two bones under the gluteal or butt muscles called the ischial tuberosities. So the patient has gone from having all of his or her weight distributed throughout the entire backside to being entirely on two bones in the butt. So where would you guess patients are going to experience discomfort when they first sit in a chair? You guessed it: the butt. The other area of discomfort upon sitting for the first few days is the low back. The muscles of the low back have performed significantly less work lying in bed for weeks. Now the patient is sitting in a chair, and those muscles have to work again to help support the spinal column in the new weight-bearing position.

The first time the patient sits in a chair following a period of being bedbound, the staff member responsible for the skin integrity (typically the nurse or a wound nurse) should be consulted, and a time limit set to avoid any type of skin breakdown.

When patients are required to be bedbound for whatever reason, there are several things that can be done, depending on the medical restrictions. If patients do not have enough strength to move their limbs on their own, a staff member can perform passive range of motion (PROM). Someone simply moves the patients' arms and legs for them. You can ask the physical therapist to teach you to perform PROM if you are visiting the patient frequently. It is very important to understand that *this does not improve the patient's strength*. It merely maintains the mobility in the joint and elasticity in the muscle. If the patient is able to move his or her limbs somewhat or has any type of active muscle contraction, staff can perform active assisted range of motion (AAROM). The patients contribute what they can to the movement, and staff assists them through the range. The goal of staff is to do as little as possible and make the patient do as much as possible. Unlike PROM, AAROM can effect strengthening as the patient is actually participating and working. With active range of motion (AROM), the patients move through a range on their own without assistance. If patients are bedbound, not confused, and able to perform AROM on their own, they can request that their physical therapist give them some AROM exercises to perform on their own between therapy sessions.

This next point is critical. Bed exercises are never a substitute for out-of-bed activities. Patients will often request bed exercises because they are easier than out-of-bed activities. Getting out of bed and mobilizing in a wheelchair is going to have significantly more carryover to functional activities, such as standing and walking, than any bed exercises. If the patient is cleared to get out of bed, this should be the priority. Once the patient is cleared for out-of-bed activity, he or she should be performing bed exercises *only* to supplement the out-of-bed activities and *not* in place of them. Again, all this should be directed by the onsite physical therapist. One of the best activities we have found for transitioning from being bedbound to being independent again is wheelchair mobility. If the patient has a seatbelt for safety, wheelchair mobility allows him or her to exercise in an upright position without significant risk of falling. This is a great activity that can be performed between therapy sessions and can build activity tolerance/endurance for quicker progression during therapy. Individual hospital policies will dictate which activities can be done. Staff can assist the patient to a chair, but, again, this is only performed with the approval of the physical therapist.

Another common misconception is that once a patient has access to therapy and an array of health-care professionals, this will fix years of inactivity and bad habits. Therapy is not magic. A patient who is overweight, who has spent the last five years smoking two packs of cigarettes a day, and whose daily mobility has included walking from the bed to the bathroom and kitchen will most likely not end up being a community ambulator. There are two primary reasons. First, physically, such patients have deconditioned their bodies/lungs/hearts to a point that it may not be possible. Second, from a motivational perspective, it is apparently not a priority for them. If it was not a priority before being hospitalized, it will most likely not be a priority during hospitalization. There are obviously exceptions to this, and there are circumstances where patients go home stronger than they were before. Generally, people's mobility and level of conditioning tends to be a product of what they are willing to actually do. Sure, there are people who are victims of terrible accidents or illnesses such as spinal cord injuries, multiple sclerosis, cerebral palsy, and so on. However, even within those illnesses, there can be a wide range of mobility depending on what the person is willing to actually do. My point is simple. What most people are willing to do in the hospital is not vastly different from what they were doing prior to admission. The people willing to push themselves prior to admission typically are the same ones who push themselves in the hospital. There is this belief sometimes that hospitalization is a wake-up call for patients. In some cases, it absolutely is. Unfortunately, it is not so for the majority. The desire of the patient can be a larger determinant to the outcome than the level of disability.

There is a range of outcomes for each individual determined by the prior level of function and the current disability. Where the patient ends up within that range is determined by his or her desire to do whatever it takes to get better. Again, notice my words "desire to do whatever it takes" and not "desire to get better." As an analogy, I think most people desire a perfectly fit, toned body. However, few have the desire to do whatever it takes to achieve that body. This dynamic does not change in a hospital environment.

In circumstances where the patient has limited desire to work hard and go home, family can encourage but cannot do the work for the patient. It is important for family members to realize their limits in this situation. If you are doing all you can to encourage the patient, you should not feel guilty.

Orthostatic hypotension is a drop in blood pressure due to a change in position. It is addressed in the next section as well for reference purposes. This is often the reason patients experience dizziness when sitting up on the edge of the bed for the first time. It is not typically a great concern other than the fact that it increases the immediate risk of falling. Usually, this will resolve after a few days of upright activity. The takeaway is to be sure to take extra time when changing positions to give the body ample opportunity to adjust to each position. There should be a staff member present for transfers until it is determined by staff that the patient is safe with mobility.

Anxiety about falling is very common among patients who have been hospitalized for an extended period. The combination of deconditioning and reorienting to upright body positioning, not to mention the increased work of the heart, gives patients a feeling that they are not in control of their bodies. The health-care providers play a big role at this point by positioning themselves directly in front of the patient (while the patient is sitting on the edge of the bed), between the patient and the floor. Next, the providers should demonstrate confidence that there will be no opportunity for a patient to fall while the provider is standing there. This encourages greater participation from the patient. The patient is responsible for listening carefully to providers and putting forth his or her best effort.

This next point is more of an aside for patients after discharge. Although it is not a perfect fit with the tenets of this manual, I have seen such incredible outcomes with the following form of therapy. It is my personal belief that this is one of the most underused forms of rehabilitation. Aquatic therapy or exercising in the pool has the benefit of allowing the buoyancy of the water to reduce the full force of gravity, which lends itself well to conditions such as osteoporosis, arthritis, back pain, and many neurological conditions. The water in many therapy pools is heated, which, again, helps with conditions such as arthritis. Many therapy pools have a chair lift in which the patient is able to sit and then be lowered into the pool if he or she is unable to walk into it. A good aquatic program will provide benefits and functional outcomes that many other programs may not. The requirements of each individual pool program may vary, but typically they require that the patient be continent and have no open wounds.

Fourteen

Orthostatic Hypotension

For patients who have been bedbound for an extended period of time, getting into an upright position and moving are critical to functional mobility. The initial positional change can cause a temporary condition called orthostatic hypotension or a temporary decrease in blood pressure due to the change in position. This can result in symptomatic dizziness. Again, this is not uncommon for patients who have been flat on their backs (supine) for a while. The reason I mention this is that it increases a patient's risk of falling due to dizziness, lightheadedness, and, in extreme cases, fainting or loss of consciousness.

Fifteen

Orthopedic Injuries

Any injuries affecting bones, muscles, tendons, or ligaments are orthopedic injuries. There are volumes of books addressing just this subject. For the purpose of this manual, I would like to stick with the most common situation that will impact the overall stay. With inpatient hospital stays, this tends to be bone fractures or broken bones. Bone fractures may require a period of limited or no weight bearing to allow them to heal properly. As a general rule, it takes six to eight weeks for bones to heal. However, there are many variables that may increase the healing time. Areas with poor blood supply or poor circulation, diabetes, and more severe fractures will all increase the healing time. Anti-inflammatory drugs and blood thinners can also negatively impact the healing process. Bone fractures can impact the patient's ability to sit, stand, or walk and ultimately the length of stay. They can also impact the discharge destination. If a patient is unable to bear weight on an extremity by the time he or she is medically stable enough for discharge, it can affect the ability to function independently at home. In this case, the patient may need to go to an intermediary facility such as an acute rehabilitation hospital or a skilled nursing facility.

Sixteen

Contracture Boots

With any prolonged hospitalization, if the patient is not able to actively move his or her ankles, the back of the calf muscles can become shortened and tight because of the way the ankle joint articulates combined with the effect of gravity. Contracture boots can be used to limit this loss of ankle flexibility. The boots typically consist of a hard plastic shell lined with a fleece or sheepskin type of material, although they can come in other forms. They maintain the ankle in a neutral position (that is, hold the ankle at a ninety-degree angle) and keep the calf muscles (gastrocnemius and soleus) stretched so that at some point if the patient is able to progress to a standing position, then loss of ankle flexibility will not be a barrier. The patient may still experience discomfort in the calves when standing for the first time after a prolonged period of being bedbound. The new demands of weight bearing and increased dorsiflexion (ankle bending in a direction with toes moving toward the shin bone) combine to create this discomfort or pain. Typically, this resolves relatively quickly with a few trials of standing, although all patients respond differently.

Seventeen

Day-Night Orientation

It is not uncommon for patients to lose orientation between day and night in the hospital. I frequently walk into a patient's room and see a completely dark and noiseless environment. I recommend, when appropriate, keeping the blinds or curtains open during the day and having some noise, maybe a little television. This does not mean turning the volume up to ten with the sun shining full force at midday on the patient. It means to be sure to have a little bit of stimulation during the day so that the patient is able to differentiate between day and night. Obviously, consult with staff regarding each individual patient before changing the room environment. There are situations where changing the environment may not be appropriate.

Eighteen

Discharge

When considering the order of topics in this book, it would seem to make more sense to place the discharge section closer to the end. However, as I will explain in greater detail below, *discharge needs to be your focus from the very beginning of the hospital stay.* One of the most stressful events for patients and families (beyond the initial admission) is discharge. I would highly suggest locating the case manager/social worker/discharge planner (each facility may have a different title for this position) as early in the stay as possible.

Ask the following questions:

- What is the average length of stay on this floor/unit?
- What are the criteria for discharge (for example, does the patient have to be walking and independent with mobility and so on)?
- Where are patients typically discharged (home, acute rehab, skilled nursing facility)?
- How much notice will I be given prior to the patient being discharged?
- Who ultimately makes the discharge decisions?

Document all answers in your journal. As the staff members answer your questions, repeat what they said back to them to prevent any misunderstandings. Use the following verbiage: "If I understand correctly, you said (repeat back to them what you believe they told you)." I outlined this technique in the section on keeping a journal. I strongly encourage you to use this method of clarification throughout the hospital stay.

It is important to understand who ultimately makes the discharge decision. The exact procedure may vary among institutions, but I will give you a general idea about the overall series of events. Typically, this is what happens. The hospitalist takes the information from all the disciplines and makes a decision on discharge. For example, the physical therapist states that the patient is safe mobility-wise to go home. The cardiologist states that the patient is safe from a cardiac standpoint. The pulmonologist clears the patient from a respiratory standpoint and so on. The hospitalist makes the ultimate decision and lets the case manager know. The hospitalist then documents in the chart that the patient is cleared for discharge based on those assessments.

However, here is a word of caution since I have seen this situation occur multiple times. There will be occasions when physicians may use imprecise language and unintentionally confuse patients and families. For example, the cardiologist may state, "The patient is safe to go home." He or she may be intending to say, "From a cardiology standpoint, the patient is safe to go home," not knowing that the patient is unsafe with mobility or that the respiratory/urology specialists have not cleared the patient for discharge, and he or she is therefore not safe to go home. Now if the patient has been cleared by all other disciplines and cardiology is the last one, the cardiologist may be accurate, but it is always best to clarify at the time with the physician and subsequently confirm with the case manager/discharge planner.

As mentioned above, from day one, you should be thinking about and focusing your questions around the eventual discharge. Do not wait until staff brings the subject up. If the plan is a discharge home, be sure to think through what each aspect of the patient's day will look like upon return home. Start with waking in the morning and address each activity that the patient will need to perform over the course of a normal day until bedtime. Here is a general idea of daily activities to think about. This list is not all inclusive:

- If you are taking the patient home in your car, does the patient need assistance in and out of the car? Are you physically able to provide that assistance?
- When the patient arrives home, are there stairs that he or she needs to manage?
- Does the patient need assistance getting out of bed?
- Does the patient need assistance getting from the bed to the toilet?
- Does he or she need assistance with toileting?
- Does the patient need assistance with meals?
- Does he or she need assistance with medication management?
- Does the patient need assistance with grocery shopping?
- Does he or she need assistance getting to physicians appointments?
- Does the patient require any equipment at home (such as a walker, wheelchair, toilet riser, shower chair, shower bars, ramp for home entrance, and so on)?
- Is the patient receiving any type of home health or outpatient services?
- Does the patient need a life alert?

It is best to get as many questions as possible answered before the day of discharge, especially in the case of a discharge home. On the day of discharge home, be certain that all of your questions have been answered. Be certain that any questions about medications, follow-up appointments with physicians, equipment being delivered, and outpatient/home health appointments are all answered.

Here's a special note to those considering being a home caregiver for a family member: Be certain to realize that in the hospital, there are multiple shifts and multiple departments pitching in to assist with all activities: toileting, medication management, transfers, and meals. Once you get home, there is one shift, one department, and one person—*you*. Be sure to thoroughly consider what this will involve. Go through the same process I discussed above. Walk through each aspect of the day mentally.

Nineteen

Patient's Valuables, Visiting Hours, and Overnight Policy

Hospital visiting hours vary from facility to facility. Some hospitals allow overnight stays if the patient is in a private room. The nurse or charge nurse should be able to give you this information.

Do not leave patient's valuables in the hospital if at all avoidable. Take them home. If the patient has expensive hearing aids, take them home as they are small, easy to lose, and may cost thousands of dollars to replace. You can purchase a small amplifier with headphones usually for around thirty dollars. If it gets lost, it is much cheaper and easier to replace. Do an online search for "FiiO portable headphone amplifier."

Twenty

Vitals

In the hospital, clinicians use a lot of different numbers to determine the patient's health. For the purpose of this manual, we are going to review just a few basic vitals numbers: temperature, respiration rate, heart rate, blood pressure, and blood oxygen level/oximetry.

*Temperature: average in adults = 98.6°F/37°C (may be slightly less than this when taken orally)

Febrile (with fever)—typically greater than 99.9 °F

*Respiration Rate: average in adults is twelve to twenty breaths per minute

- Tachypnea—greater than twenty breaths per minute
- Apnea—cessation of breathing (sleep apnea is a common condition in which breathing ceases for a period during sleep)
- Dyspnea—shortness of breath (SOB) can be exertional (following exercise)

*Heart Rate: normal in adults = sixty to one hundred beats per minute

- Tachycardia—greater than one hundred beats per minute
- Bradycardia—less than sixty beats per minute

*Blood Pressure: the upper number is called systolic; the lower number is called diastolic
- Normal = <120/<80
- Orthostatic = <90/<60
- Hypertensive = >139/>89 = greater risk for stroke or heart attack

*Oximetry: oxygen saturation of blood
- Normal = 95–99 percent
- Normal for someone with COPD = 88–94 percent

Other numbers not covered here are labs, which are run on a patient at the physician's discretion. This is a blood test that provides further values and gives clinicians more information and insight into what is happening with the patient medically. Covering this subject is a book in and of itself. The physician or nurse can quickly review the patient's lab results with you, highlighting any areas of concern.

Another blood test specific to the respiratory system is an arterial blood gas (ABG), which gives insight into how the respiratory system is moving oxygen and carbon dioxide.

Twenty-One

Hospital-Acquired Infection and Infection Control

The most important technique to prevent the spread of infection is good hand hygiene. Hand washing and using/changing of gloves between patient contacts by staff are the best ways to protect patients. Make sure staff members who come in contact with the patient are practicing good hygiene.

Some common infections seen in hospitals are methicillin-resistant staphylococcus auras (MRSA), clostridium difficile colitis (C-diff), vancomycin-resistant enterococcus (VRE), acinetobacter, and klebsiella. Depending on hospital policy, there may be additional measures to prevent the spread of such organisms such as the mandatory use of gown, gloves, and masks by staff and visitors when patients are found to have these infections. Each hospital will have its own policy. Check with your nurse or charge nurse if this is applicable. Usually, there will be a sign outside the patient's room notifying visitors of the additional precautions.

Twenty-Two

Deep Vein Thrombosis

One of the risks for patients who lack mobility is called a deep vein thrombosis (DVT). This is a type of blood clot. Patients are at an increased risk for DVT when they are immobile. Anticoagulant medications (blood thinners) and compression pumps can be used to reduce the risk of DVTs. Compression pumps are sleeves typically with Velcro securement that are applied around the calves, attached to a pump, and intermittently inflated and deflated to move the blood in the lower legs when the patient is unable to move his or her legs actively. DVT is also mentioned in the changes in status section above.

Twenty-Three

Medical Power of Attorney /
Release of Information

Medical information about the patient is released only to family unless the patient or designate (this is the medical power of attorney if one has been appointed) consents to its release to others. The Health Insurance Portability and Accountability Act (HIPAA) of 1996 governs how health-care providers can use personal health information (PHI). In other words, HIPAA dictates how health-care providers handle patient privacy.

Twenty-Four

Most Common Lines (Tubes Attached to the Patient)

When you walk into a hospital room, especially an intensive care unit (ICU) or any unit housing patients who are very sick, there will oftentimes be a multitude of lines (wires/tubes) attached to the patient. The following list is not comprehensive but will give you a general idea and a starting point for asking questions. I have broken it down by body function to help you relate it to daily life and to make it easier to understand.

Eating:
- A percutaneous endoscopic gastrostomy (PEG) tube is surgically inserted through the abdomen to feed the patient.
- A duotube is run into the nose down the esophagus and into the stomach.
- Total parenteral nutrition (TPN) is nutrition run through an intravenous (IV) line.

Urinating:
- A Foley catheter for men or women is inserted through the urethra and into the bladder, has a bag attached to collect the urine, and is easily identifiable.

Breathing:
- Ventilator: If the patient is unable to breathe on his or her own, a tube can be inserted through the mouth *or* through a surgical opening in the front of the neck (tracheostomy).
- Supplemental oxygen: If the patient is able to breathe on his or her own but is not getting enough oxygen into the bloodstream, oxygen can be run through a nasal cannula or tube that typically rests on both ears and has an outlet dispensing oxygen into the nose.
- Oximetry: Usually a probe is attached to the finger or toe (occasionally the ear or forehead) that measures the percentage of oxygen in the blood (see vitals section).

Medication:
- Peripheral lines—inserted into veins of forearms and feet.
- Central lines—generally inserted in neck, chest, or groin.
- Peripherally inserted central catheter (PICC) lines—generally inserted in upper arm.

Heart:
- Telemetry: Usually three to five sticky pads placed around the patient's chest that monitor the cardiac (heart) rate and rhythm.

The decision about which feeding and medication mechanisms to be used will depend on individual factors.

Please keep in mind that with all the machines and monitors in the room, there are inevitably going to be alarms sounding from time to time. Do not panic. There are multiple reasons for alarms to sound. In some cases, it can be as simple as a poor connection. Contact the nurse and ask him/her to explain what is happening.

Twenty-Five

Depression

It is very common for patients to exhibit symptoms of depression in the hospital. This can affect willingness to participate in therapy, eating habits, and many of the activities that contribute to a quick and full recovery. My personal opinion is that this is an often undertreated issue. As an example, the effect of depression on a patient's willingness to participate in physical therapy can be profound. If you are concerned about this issue, speak with the nurse or case manager. Ask if there is a psychologist or psychiatrist who has privileges on the unit.

A psychologist cannot prescribe medications, whereas a psychiatrist can. Psychologists can recommend medications to the physician, who can in turn prescribe those medications if he or she feels it is appropriate. Be very careful and outline exactly what your expectations are before any medications are added. For example, if the patient is a new amputee and is depressed, prescribing a medication to improve mood may be appropriate if determined so by the physician. However, is that a long-term solution to a new permanent problem? It is important that the underlying issue be addressed and not just medicated. If medication is determined to be appropriate, ask the physician and do your own research regarding potential side effects. Let me be very clear in that I am not advocating that the patient be medicated in this situation. I am merely stating that if depression is a possible issue, it should not be ignored. Again, this is determined by the physician, but you should be involved and ask questions.

There are support groups in the community for many types of patient populations. A few examples are amputee, brain injury, and stroke support groups. I strongly encourage patients and family members to reach out to people who have gone through similar situations. Often, people who have been through or are going through the same events as the patient are able to reach him or her in a way that family or health-care providers are not.

Twenty-Six

Family Members Need to Take Care of Their Own Health as Well

It is important for you as a family member to recognize that your health is critical. Going to the hospital daily and spending long hours there can have negative consequences over the course of a long hospitalization. It is important to get out of the hospital to sleep and take care of your personal responsibilities. If you make yourself sick, how are you going to take care of the patient? Taking care of yourself is truly the best thing you can do for the patient. It is necessary to have a long-term view. Do not feel guilty about taking the time to take care of yourself. This guilt is very common. If you are afraid to leave due to concern about missing the doctor, leave your telephone number with the nurse and request a call.

Twenty-Seven

Respiratory Issues/
Ventilator

A ventilator is a machine that performs or assists with the activity of breathing for a patient when he or she is unable to breathe on his or her own. It is not uncommon for people with compromised respiratory systems not to have enough strength to breathe on their own following surgical procedures that require anesthesia. In addition, following severe trauma such as a motor vehicle accident, a ventilator may be necessary until the patient regains respiratory strength.

The ventilator is used when the respiratory muscles are too weak and require assistance. This is distinguished from supplemental oxygen, which is dispensed through a tube (nasal cannula) that attaches to an oxygen source on one end and typically has an outlet into the patient's nose. In this case, the patient has enough strength in the respiratory muscles to support breathing independently but is not getting enough oxygen into the bloodstream. Adding supplemental oxygen increases the concentration of oxygen that the patient is breathing and thus increases the amount of oxygen that makes it into the bloodstream.

A person is attached to a ventilator in one of two ways. The first is oral intubation, where a breathing tube is inserted in the patient's mouth and down into the trachea. The second is via a tracheostomy. In this procedure, a surgical incision is made in the lower front of the neck through which a tube is inserted directly into the trachea. This is called a tracheostomy or trach tube. Staff will often refer to this simply as "the trach." In both cases, a tube is inserted into the trachea in which to provide pressure and assist the patient with the mechanics of breathing. The difference is merely the entry point of the tube.

The decision to intubate orally or perform a tracheostomy is typically dependent on the length of time a patient is expected to be on a ventilator. Oral intubation may be more appropriate for shorter time periods, while longer periods may necessitate a tracheostomy. Patients who are in need of chronic ventilation may have a tracheostomy performed. Regarding oral intubation, it is important to know that trauma can occur to the trachea and vocal cords in the process of inserting the tube. When the tube is removed, there may be residual speech and swallowing issues that require the skills of a speech language pathologist (speech therapist).

Being on a ventilator is typically not a permanent condition. In the majority of cases, patients can be transitioned off the ventilator through a process called ventilator weaning. In this scenario, the amount of support or pressure that the ventilator is supplying is slowly decreased, while the respiratory muscles are gradually allowed to do more and more work. Analogous to working out with weights and steadily increasing the weight, in this situation the respiratory muscles are slowly doing more work until they are hopefully able to support independent breathing. The ability to wean and the speed at which a patient is able to be weaned from the ventilator depend on many factors. One of these is the health of the lungs prior to admission. Everything else being equal, a heavy cigarette smoker is going to have much more difficulty being weaned from the ventilator than a marathon runner. Sedative medications can depress the respiratory system and slow the weaning process.

This is a very rudimentary explanation of a very complex process. There are a myriad of situations that may occur. Therefore, any questions regarding this process should be discussed with the pulmonologist and respiratory therapists.

Two of the more common questions asked by patients weaning from the ventilator are:

1. When can I eat?
2. When can I talk?

The answers to these questions are highly individual. Obviously, if the patient is orally intubated (tube through the mouth), the endotracheal tube will need to be removed first. In the case of someone with a trach tube, it will depend on several factors, including the individual hospital policy. In regard to talking for a patient with a tracheostomy, if the patient has been weaned from the ventilator and is able to breathe on his or her own, generally the pulmonologist will decide when it is appropriate to attempt to use a Passy-Muir valve (PMV). This is a one-way (air comes in but not out) valve that is placed over the tracheostomy, allowing the patient to speak. Decisions about swallowing/eating are generally made by the pulmonologist in collaboration with the speech language pathologist (SLP)/speech therapist.

Twenty-Eight

Listen to Your Loved One

It is important to take time and determine what the patient truly wants. There are occasions when families believe they know better than the patient what is best. In some instances, the patient's cognitive abilities while in the hospital are not indicative of his or her usual state (that is, in the hospital, he or she may experience confusion/disorientation). This is a good example of a situation in which the family can take a larger role in the decision-making process. However, I have seen situations in which the families of patients who had just weeks to live advocated for multiple procedures and aggressive therapy that made the patient's final weeks of life less than comfortable. I am not advocating a position here. If this is what the patient would have truly wanted, then the family members are just acting as good advocates. I am merely attempting to provide a full perspective. The bottom line is to be certain to take the time to have a serious discussion with your loved ones and listen to their views and desires. Ultimately, you are the patient advocate, so be certain to accurately represent what the patient wants.

Twenty-Nine

Circulation

This section is included to help clarify one of many reasons recovery time varies among patients. To oversimplify slightly, the body heals itself with nutrients from the blood. The circulation and supply of blood to injured areas are often primary factors in recovery time. Any condition or activity that affects circulation can affect recovery time. Any circulatory diseases, such as peripheral artery disease (PAD), peripheral vascular disease (PVD), arteriosclerosis, and diabetes (to name just a few), can delay the healing process. Smoking and diabetes can also affect the circulatory system, which in turn affects the body's ability to heal itself. Simply, all other factors being equal, better circulation generally equates to quicker healing time.

Thirty

Avoiding Hospitalization

I debated about whether to include this section. Ultimately, I decided it was good information and should be included, especially given recent trends and the skyrocketing costs of health care. Illness in many cases has multifactorial causes, including congenital factors, environmental factors, and age. However, there are a disproportionate number of hospitalizations due to smoking, diabetes, and obesity. These issues can be the primary cause of illness or contributing factors. They also tend to complicate or prolong the recovery time. People who are healthier tend to have more infrequent hospitalizations and shorter hospital stays (all other factors being equal). Of course, bad things happen to healthy people all the time. However, in general, you have a degree of control over your own health. I don't say this to be judgmental. I say this because there seems to be a lack of awareness of the significant role that lifestyle can play in hospitalizations. I am not advocating that you begin marathon training or a raw food regimen tomorrow. I am only suggesting that if you smoke, if you are significantly overweight, or if your activity level consists of moving as little as possible, there is a strong possibility this may impact your future health. You don't need to be a pulmonologist to realize that if you smoke and you become sick, your chances of ending up on a ventilator are significantly greater than someone who does not smoke. If you are overweight, can barely walk short distances, and end up falling and breaking a hip, then your chances of ending up in a care center for a couple of months while that leg heals is significantly greater than for someone in good shape who can stand and walk with crutches. Some people take illness and hospitalization as a sign that health needs to be a greater priority. Ultimately, what is more important in life than your health? It is difficult to fully enjoy family, friends, work, and many of life's other joys from a hospital bed.

Thirty-One

Online Research and References

Using the Internet has changed the amount of information we have access to at any given time and the speed at which we can access it. It is a tool that can help patients and families better understand medical conditions and procedures. The downside is the potential for misinformation. Here is the catch-22: most websites that are easier to understand tend to be less directed toward health-care professionals and therefore can be less reliable. The more reliable websites tend to be more difficult to read, have more medical terminology, and be more difficult to traverse. If the truth be told, if I am in a hurry and need to find something quickly, I am likely to use Wikipedia. Just be aware that anything you find on the Internet may have limited reliability. It is best to consider the source of the site. If the source is a physician group, health-care organization, government, or any group solely devoted to health care, the information will tend to be more accurate. In addition, *looking up a few facts on the Internet does not give you the ability to diagnose illness*. As stated earlier, this is just a starting point for discussion with the professionals. I have included a few sites that might be helpful in getting your feet wet.

- Medication: the specific drug-manufacturer website for that medication, PDR.net
- General information about illnesses: CDC.gov, WebMD

- Orthopedic issues: Wheelessonline.com
- Specific diseases: cancer.org, diabetes.org, heart.org

I am an advocate of patients and families doing online research, as it can provide a starting point for discussions and often lead to very specific and insightful questions.

Conclusion

I sincerely hope this manual provided you with the information needed to better manage your hospital experience. It is my goal to assist patients and families through one of the most stressful events in life. To that end, I need your assistance. Please e-mail me at hospital-survivalguide@gmail.com and provide feedback. Let me know specifically which sections in this manual you found to be particularly helpful. Please also identify any information not included that would have been of value to you. This way, I can continually improve this manual and provide the most current, comprehensive, and useful information to help future patients and families. Your feedback is invaluable. Thank you for allowing me to assist you on your journey. Best wishes to you and your family for a happy and healthy life.

About the Author

Ronald Wild is a physical therapist with nineteen years' experience. He has worked in multiple settings including inpatient acute care, outpatient, long-term acute care (LTACH), acute rehabilitation, and skilled nursing. This includes staff and managerial positions. He holds bachelors of science degrees from the University of Buffalo in physical therapy and business administration. He is currently functional movement screen (FMS) certified and a previously certified strength and conditioning specialist (CSCS).